DEDICATION

This handbook is dedicated to all the amazing families, friends, and formal care partners who so caringly support individuals who are living with dementia on their unexpected journeys. You are inspirational!

ACKNOWLEDGMENTS

We gratefully acknowledge and thank Jackie Pinkowitz, Jan Bays, Nancy Kriseman and Barbara Leipow for their talented editing of the handbook.

With gratitude to Karen Love who guided the development of this handbook from concept through publication with unwavering dedication and inspiration.

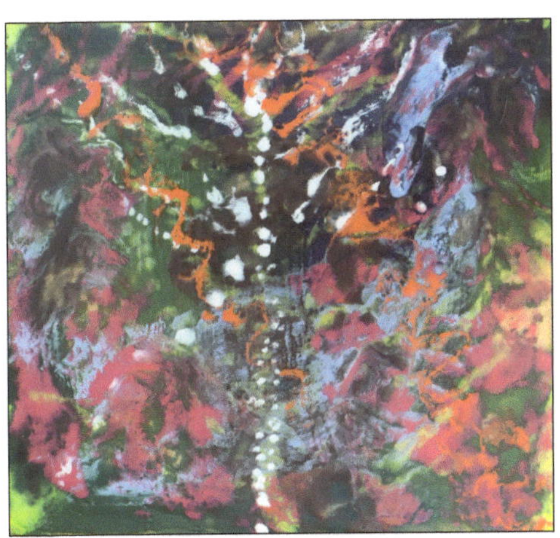

Garden Tree
Encaustic, 2016 • Carol Ambrogio Wood

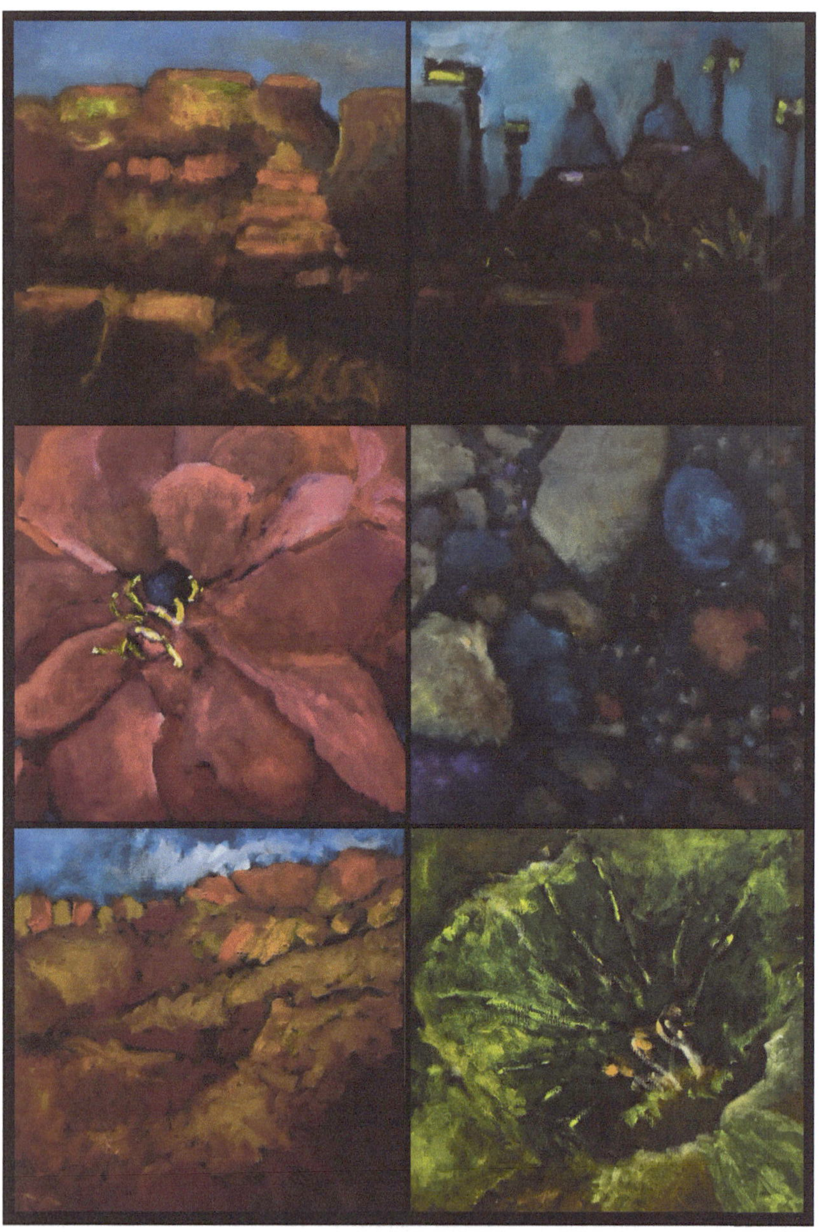

*Yellow Flower (2016), Stones (2016), Spires (2016),
Plateau (2015), Red Flower (2016), Canyon (2015)*
Oil on canvas • Tony Shopinski

FORWARD

There are many resources available about the cognitive changes and impairments associated with dementia, including Alzheimer's. Little has been written, however, about LIVING with, what for many will be, a long-term condition. This handbook provides information and insights provided by people living with dementia and their care partners to help family and friends better understand living with early and moderate symptoms of dementia, and how to best support someone you care about. The Dementia Action Alliance is developing a separate care partner handbook for advanced symptoms of dementia.

The typical focus on the degenerative aspects of dementia fuels stigmatizing behaviors and practices that add to the isolation, fear and challenges of living with dementia.

"We are so much more than our diseased brain! We each have a unique personality that will shine through. We can draw on our inner resources to cope with this new challenge — with your help and encouragement."

— Christine Bryden, with permission from "Nothing About Us, Without Us?," p 61.

Baby boomers and younger generations of people currently living with dementia are speaking out about wanting to live purposeful lives with dementia. While dementia is indeed a challenging condition, there are many ways to help someone live productively with it.

> *"I can't pass as the Old Me anymore.*
> *That's clear. So today I stop trying. Today, I start to enjoy the New Me. I can still learn, teach, risk, love, fail and try. And as I evolve with my dementia, I'll surely do things differently. I'll just have to figure out my new role in society. I still have the right to enjoy life, and I still want to make a difference.*
>
> *— Mary Radnowsky, with permission from "One. It Can Be Everything."*

Dementia is a companion condition; it affects not only the person who has it, but also his or her family and friends. You unexpectedly are along on a journey of caring that will be unique to you and the person in your life with dementia. While it is not a chosen journey, with a positive and proactive outlook and attitude, it can be a time filled with joy, humor, achievement, and love.

The **Resources** section in the back of the handbook provides information about additional materials that can be helpful to care partners.

Table of Contents

What is Dementia?

Like cancer, dementia is an umbrella term that includes
many different forms of dementia. The most common form
is Alzheimer's disease. Other common forms are vascular
dementia, Lewy Body dementia, frontotemporal dementia
and mixed dementia (a combination of several forms
of dementia). Dementia describes a group of cognitive
symptoms such as difficulty remembering, concentrating or
problem-solving; shortened attention span, confusion with
location or the passage of time; impairments in judgement,
word-finding, and learning; and changes in behavior and
social abilities.[1]

Dementia has no boundaries. It affects men and women,
people of all ethnicities, income and educational levels.
Although dementia is more common in older adults, it is not
a part of normal aging. Individuals younger than age 65
can be affected. In the United States, it is estimated that
over 200,000 people younger than age 65 are living
with dementia.

The symptoms and the progression of dementia vary
depending on the form. Some forms of dementia progress
slowly over years, while other forms such as vascular
dementia may result in the sudden loss of some cognitive
functions.

Often people do not recognize the changes in themselves.
Others who have regular contact with them notice the

---

[1] See the Mayo Clinic's website for more information — http://www.mayoclinic.
org/ diseases- conditions/dementia/basics/definition/con-20034399 .

changes first. The adage, "Ignorance is bliss," may be useful for some things in life but it is not an advisable strategy for one's health. If a person is exhibiting some changed cognitive symptoms, it is important to be assessed by a physician. The symptoms may be a result of other conditions that are treatable such as thyroid problems, vitamin B-12 deficiency, reactions to a medication, infections, and depression among other possibilities.

It is important to know that not all physicians have expertise in assessing and diagnosing dementia, and some that do are not comfortable delivering a dementia diagnosis. This is generally because there currently are no cures for any forms of dementia and there are very limited treatment options.

For some people, how the diagnosis of dementia was delivered can add to the trauma of learning they have a chronic, degenerative health condition. Often individuals are told they need to put their affairs in order and return in six months to monitor the progression. It is the exceptional physician who provides information and encouragement about continuing to live one's life fully and purposefully with dementia.

Having proactive information at the time of diagnosis is vitally important and beneficial as this is a key window of time when perceptions and expectations about living with dementia are being formed. This handbook provides you with the proactively oriented information that otherwise may be hard to find.

Grief is Normal and Natural

Learning that your spouse, a family member or close friend has dementia can feel like a sucker punch. That is a normal human reaction to life altering news. You may experience a wide range of emotions including numbness, denial, sadness, guilt, anger, anxiety, helplessness, frustration and blame. These symptoms of grief are a normal and natural reaction.

Grief is an individualized process with no set time frame as it is unique for each individual. It is important to allow yourself to experience grief in order to move beyond it. Knowing what to expect along the grieving process can be helpful. Dr. Elisabeth Kubler-Ross's famous stages of grief are a useful general guide[2]. The stages are not linear or predictable, and they may occur in any order, if at all.

- Denial — Being unable or unwilling to accept your loved one or close friend has dementia. It may feel as though you are experiencing a bad dream and are waiting to "wake up" so things will be back to normal.

- Anger — Feeling angry that he or she has dementia and the unfairness of it.

- Bargaining — Pleading to a higher power to undo or reverse the condition.

---

[2] Retrieved online on November 2, 2016, http://www.ekrfoundation.org/five-stages-of-grief/.

- Depression — Feeling a range of emotions and behaviors such as sadness, irritability, guilt, sleep too little or too much, change in eating habits, withdrawal from people and activities.

- Acceptance — Accepting the condition, you are able to re-engage in daily life.

This is a time to be especially gentle and patient with yourself. You may want to confide in one or more trusted friends about how you are feeling so that your emotions don't bottle up inside you. Seeking professional support, such as through a therapist or psychologist, is another helpful option. You can also check online to see if there is a Memory Café or Early-Stage Care Partner chat group near you.

Suggestions

♦ Be kind and gentle with yourself.

♦ Confide in a close family member or friend. There is truth in the adage, "A sorrow shared is a sorrow halved."

♦ Do things that fill your soul such as nature walks, spend time with people you are close to — do what makes you feel better.

♦ Participate in an online café and talk with others living with dementia — http://www.dementiaalliance international.org/events/cafe-le-brain/.

Telling Others You Have Dementia

Because of the stigma associated with having dementia, many people are not comfortable telling others their loved one or close friend has dementia. The downside is that the silence adds to the closeted nature of living with dementia. Fortunately, there is a cultural shift underway as baby boomers and younger generations of people impacted by dementia are publicly speaking out.

It's important to talk with your loved one or friend about what each of your comfort levels are about telling others. It's a valuable conversation to have jointly so you understand and respect each other's perspectives. One husband and wife decided to wait six months before telling their children. They wanted time to get used to changes in their lives, and to be able to talk with their children without becoming overly emotional.

Comfort in confiding with others about dementia aligns with a person's personality type and age. Some people are naturally open and comfortable sharing information freely while others are more guarded and only want to tell immediate family members and close friends.

> *"Does it hurt to have dementia asked my friend. Mostly it hurts inside because I can't accomplish the things I want to and I know it is not going to get better. But right now is a good moment, so let's laugh, take pictures and count our blessings for every moment we can share."*
>
> — Laurie Scherrer, with permission from Love & Laughter Blog

Common Misperceptions about Dementia

When a person's network of family, friends, neighbors, health care providers, and local community members hold misperceptions about dementia, it can significantly and negatively impact everyday life. Misperceptions about dementia signal a lack of knowledge and understanding about the condition, and lead to stigmatizing attitudes and behaviors even among medical professionals.

Richard Taylor, diagnosed with early onset Alzheimer's disease at the age of 58, was one of the first Americans living with dementia to speak out publicly and widely about his experience with stigma and how damaging it was to his emotional and social well-being.

> *"Family and friends questioned my ability to make everyday decisions — Can I be trusted to spend time alone with my granddaughter? Can I, should I handle my own money, answer the door... Friends stopped calling me and when I asked why was told, 'I don't know what to say.' I said, just say hello."*
>
> — Richard Taylor, PhD (Dupuis et al, 2011[3])

---

[3] Dupuis, S.L., Wiersma, E., & Loisells, L. (2012). *Pathologizing behavior: Meanings of behaviours in dementia care.* Journal of Aging Studies, 26(2), 162-173.

There are many misperceptions about dementia. A common concern voiced by people living with early to moderate symptoms of dementia is they are often treated by others as if they had advanced symptoms of dementia. This likely is because of the media's focus on advanced symptoms of dementia leaving people with the impression that is what all dementia is like. As a result, most people don't understand the spectrum and progression of dementia and ascribe advanced symptoms to everyone living with dementia regardless of his or her symptoms. The following are other common misperceptions about living with dementia.

Misperceptions	Facts
Everyone with dementia is the same.	Every person is a unique individual. People may have some similar dementia characteristics in the same way that people with brown hair share a similar characteristic.
People who have dementia are an empty shell.	This statement indicates a lack of understanding about dementia and fuels stigmatizing behaviors and practices. Being considered an empty shell is insulting and dehumanizing. People retain their personhood and individuality lifelong including with dementia.

Misperceptions	Facts
If you can speak for yourself, you don't have dementia.	This statement also signals lack of understanding about dementia and is insulting to those who are living with dementia. Besides the fact that there are many forms of dementia, people who have early to moderate dementia symptoms are very capable of speaking for themselves. People with advanced symptoms may lose some speaking capacity, but can continue to express themselves non-verbally.
If a person has trouble finding words, they also have trouble following a conversation.	Word retrieval and expressing language are controlled by a different part of the brain than receptive language ability.
People who have dementia cannot learn new things.	The brain has vast neural reserves and with stimulating triggers can form some new neural pathways resulting in learning.

Living with Dementia

Until recently little had been written about the actual experience of living with dementia. Thanks to the global nature of the Internet and a generation of people who are comfortable using it, people living with early and moderate symptoms of dementia all over the world are writing about their experiences in blogs and online forums. Their diverse personal writings provide an expansive window into learning about living with dementia from the first person account.

> *"Here is what I wish someone had told me about three weeks after I was diagnosed. Dementia is not a death sentence. It is a wakeup call to live your life, today and every day for the rest of your life as fully as possible. You are not fading away, you are changing."*
>
> — Richard Taylor

Dementia impairs some cognitive abilities but it does not impair all abilities nor does it take away a person's humanity. Family and friends may not realize they have begun treating the individual with dementia as only their DEMENTIA rather than as a person who has a neurocognitive degenerative health condition along with all the other aspects of his or her humanness. For instance, Joyce was diagnosed with dementia at age 64. For 30 years, Joyce was a beloved teacher. Now she has very little short-term memory, but continues to enjoy reading, going to concerts and plays, and treasures visits from past students. The cognitive impairments are only one aspect of Joyce.

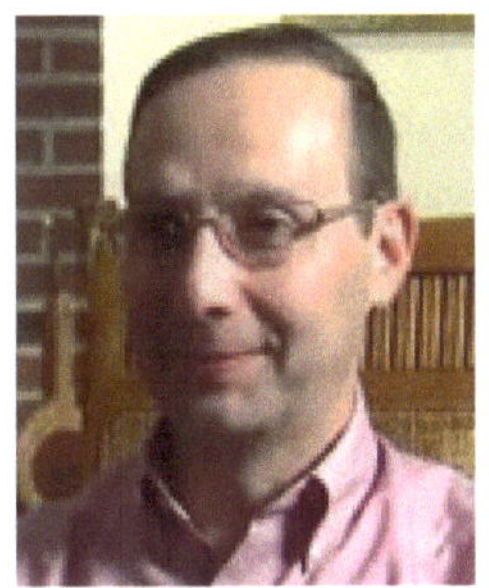

Michael Ellenbogen, a former corporate executive living with younger onset Alzheimer's, is a vocal self-advocate. Michael experienced a night and day difference in how friends and colleagues treated him before and after his dementia diagnosis.

> *"All of a sudden neighbors looked askance when I mowed the lawn, and former colleagues stopped calling to get together. I lost words, not my mind."*
>
> — Michael Ellenbogen, with permission

Christine Bryden describes her experience —

> *"The day before my diagnosis, I was a busy and successful divorced mother of three girls with a high-level job with the Australian government. The day after, I was a label – Person with Dementia. No one knew what to say, what to expect of me, how to talk to me and whether to even visit me. I had become a labelled person, defined by my disease overnight. My first two years (post-diagnosis) were a struggle of living a life transformed by this label of dementia. I felt shame and retreated from society."*
>
> — Christine Bryden, with permission from "Nothing About Us, Without Us!" p. 54.

Steven Sabat, PhD, a noted neuropsychologist from Georgetown University, describes the losses experienced by people who have dementia as not only due to the effects of their condition, but also to the psychological and emotional effects of how they are treated by others. Kate Swaffer, who was diagnosed at the age of 49 with younger onset frontotemporal dementia in 2008, gave this dynamic a name – Prescribed Disengagement®. Kate uses this term to describe what it feels like when people diagnosed with dementia are expected not to have a life and to give up.

> *"It sets us up to believe there is no hope, there are no strategies to manage the symptoms of dementia, and more importantly, that it's not worthwhile trying to find any…It also takes away any power or control of the person diagnosed, giving it all to the care partners… It has the potential to completely disable us emotionally, leading us to learned helplessness… Dementia is the only terminal illness I know of where people are told to go home and give up."*
>
> — Kate Swaffer, with permission[4]

Imagine if Prescribed Disengagement® was how Stephen Hawking was treated when he was diagnosed with early onset amyotrophic lateral sclerosis at the age of 21? He placed no limits on himself and went on to a stellar career in physics, astrology, cosmology and mathematics.

---

[4] Swaffer, K. (2016). *What the Hell Happened to My Brain? Living Beyond Dementia.* Jessica Kingsley Publishers, London, p. 160–161.

Currently, at age 75, Dr. Hawking is the Director of Research at the Centre of Theoretical Cosmology at the University of Cambridge. Kate, like Stephen Hawking, has grit and determination and placed no limits on herself. Since being diagnosed with dementia, Kate, with the support of the University's Disability Services, has earned two Bachelor degrees, a Master's of Science in Dementia Care and is currently pursuing a PhD.

Richard Taylor and Kate Swaffer among many others living with dementia believe dementia should be treated as a disability. A disability orientation focuses on what strategies and accommodations are needed so the individuals can continue to function as well as possible in their own way.

> *"I need your help to enable me,*
> *not further disable me."*
>
> — Richard Taylor

Suggestions

- Adopt an open-minded attitude and a positive approach to living with dementia as a disability which does NOT take away one's personhood or abilities.

- Focus on enabling your loved one or friend to live the best life possible.

◆ Help him/her learn to use adaptive strategies to ease daily living such as using a smart phone to send reminders.

◆ Encourage your loved one or friend to continue to engage in things that are meaningful to him or her.

◆ Smile and laugh often together.

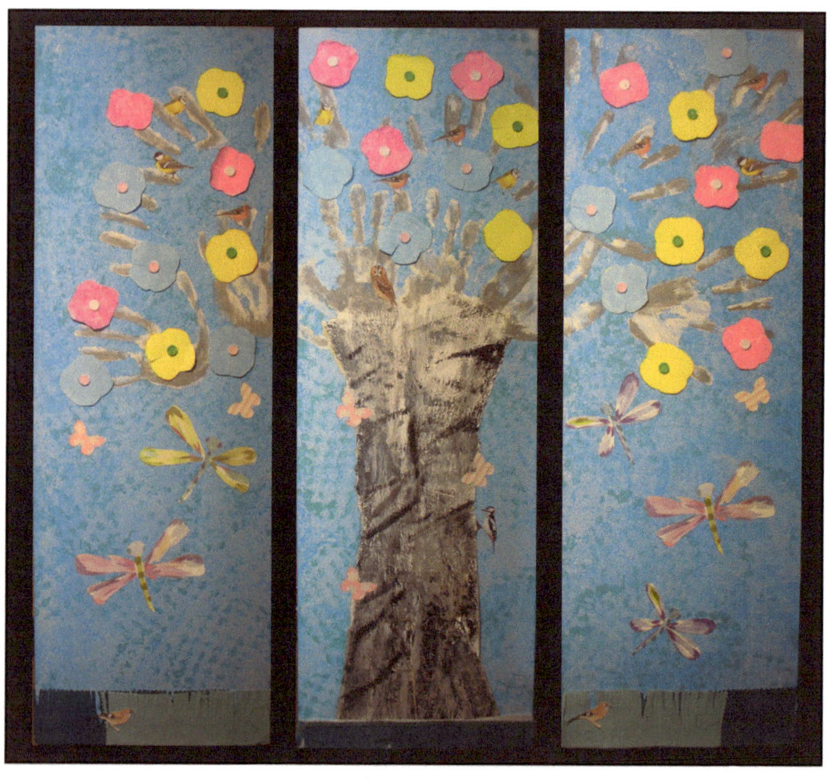

Blossom Tree
Mixed media, 2015–2016
Collaborative – Residents of Springwood Residential Home

Well-Being — A Newfound Friend

Up until now, you likely haven't given much thought to actively supporting your well-being or the well-being of your loved one or close friend. Generally, people think of well-being in terms of physical health, but well-being is broader and includes social, emotional, and spiritual dimensions as well as physical.

The "Preamble to the Constitution of the World Health Organization" defines well-being as — *A state of complete physical, mental and social well-being and not merely the absence of disease or infirmity.*

All dimensions of well-being are vital and important. Well-being is fundamental to the quality of one's life. Think about a time when you were at odds with someone important in your life and how it made you feel. You probably felt OK physically, but emotionally you may not have been OK which affected your overall sense of well-being. There are many ways well-being can be disrupted including not feeling personally safe or financially secure.

As noted already but worth repeating, most people haven't given much thought to their well-being up until now. As a care partner of a person you care about who has dementia, you will need to be mindful of your well-being. It will require active work on your part and does not naturally occur. The good news is the rewards far outweigh the effort!

It's important to stay socially, physically, emotionally and spiritually active lifelong. There is a natural tendency to let up on activity as one gets older and, more so, if facing a disabling condition. Letting up on activity is not a good choice because weakening any dimension of well-being has a cascading effect that weakens all dimensions. For instance, if a person withdraws socially, this affects the human need to connect with others and impacts them emotionally. The isolation also affects physical movement and limits the ability to keep one's body limber, flexible and strong.

A ROADMAP TO MAINTAINING YOUR WELL-BEING

- Keep your spirits up

- Develop and maintain a caring support network

- Limit stressful experiences as much as possible

- Seek fun and interesting experiences

- Expose yourself to laughter and humor

- Be open-minded to creative strategies

- Eat and drink healthily

- Learn good sleeping habits if you don't have them already

- Be physically active

- Increase opportunities to fill your spiritual soul

Fostering Well-Being Through Person-Center Practices

It is important to focus on an individual's strengths and abilities rather than on their impairments and aspects they may no longer manage well. Proactive person-centered practices enhance the quality of life for the individual who is living with dementia as well as for those who care about them. Focusing on the 'whole person' and not just his/her dementia is the difference between helping them live fully with a health condition as opposed to the health condition becoming the person's life. A focus on the 'whole person' is known as person-centered practices.

Person-centered practices enhance overall well-being because of the attention to all aspects of humanness — emotional, social, physical and spiritual. Person-centered practices can be transformative. The following communication from a friend who is living with dementia is an example of

---

[5] Sabat, S. (2011). *Flourishing of the self while caring for a person with dementia: A case study of education, counseling, and psychosocial support via email.* Dementia: The International Journal of Social Research and Practice, 10(1):81-97.

the transformative and valuable effects of person-centered practices —

> *"The two of you have changed my life.*
>
> *— You have given me purpose.*
>
> *— You have given me a reason to get up every day.*
>
> *— You have given me life after diagnosis.*
>
> *I don't know where or how to begin to say THANK YOU, so I will just say…*
>
> *THANK YOU & I LOVE YOU BOTH!"*

Person-centered practices involve a focus on all dimensions of well-being — physical, emotional, social, and spiritual.

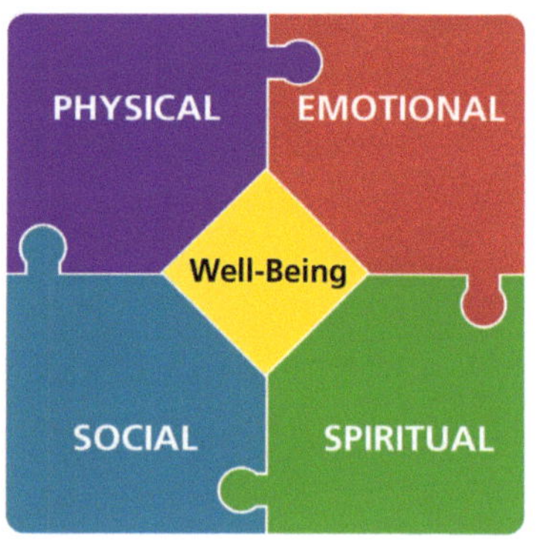

The spiritual dimension is intended here in a broad context and not as 'religion.' While participation in a religion may be a meaningful way to experience spirituality for some, spirituality does not have to involve a deity or a higher power. It is feeling deeply connected to something larger than ourselves such as nature or being of service to others. There are many other ways such as walks in nature, service to others, enjoying the arts and music, seeing a sunset, meditation, and spending time in a special place are among the experiences that enable people to feel deeply connected to something larger than themselves. As such, spirituality represents an important aspect of well-being.

All dimensions are essential and important to support well-being. Emotional, social and spiritual well-being is connected to doing things in daily life that provide routine, meaning, and purpose; bring comfort and enjoyment; and generate a sense of pride and self-worth. These human needs do not change for an individual living with dementia. What can change is the individual's ability to self-initiate activities if there is neural damage in the part of the brain that controls those functions. A common mistake care partners make is to think the individual isn't interested in doing things because they are not initiating the activity. If you are not already, you will need to become a keen observer so you can identify changed abilities and functions.

As a care partner, you can help the individual maintain activities that enhance their emotional, social and spiritual well-being. There is a line, however, between supporting individuals so they can 'help themselves' and doing things for them. Being overly 'helpful' has an unintended consequence of diminishing the individual's independence and person-hood. They need assistance setting things up, then the time and encouragement so they can do whatever they are able to manage. As a care partner it can be a gentle dance at times supporting their independence and personhood. Paradoxically, taking the time to help someone living with dementia experience successes strengthens your own sense of well-being and feelings of self-worth.

Person-Centered Practices

1 Focus on the individual's strengths and existing abilities and be realistic about what he or she can and cannot do or manage. For instance, someone who is a night owl won't be as effective doing things early in the morning.

2 Think about the person and what brings him or her comfort. This information will guide you to try things that are likely to be well received.

3 Consider activities and interests that are normal and customary for the individual such as a morning cup of coffee, walking the family dog, sitting in the garden.

4 Recognize that identifying engaging things to do takes a "trial and error" mentality. Not everything you try will work. Sometimes an activity works one day and not another.

5 Think outside the box. At 97 years old, Mary Axleroad loved using a music-painting app on an iPad. Mary's daughter, knowing her mother's love of music and art, decided to give the iPad a try with a "nothing ventured, nothing gained" spirit.

6 Be enthusiastic and encouraging. Had Mary's daughter presented the iPad initially with hesitation and a lack of encouragement, her mother likely would not have tried the iPad. HOW you present things matters.

7 Praise is valued at any age. Watch someone's eyes light up when you offer praise — "That art piece you made is amazing!"

8 Adopt a "no wrong way" spirit. People living with dementia may do tasks and use items in non-customary ways, or they may take longer to do an activity. It is OK if a person enjoys stacking puzzle pieces instead of piecing them together. Success is defined as fun and engagement.

When an individual feels cared about and has a positive sense of well-being, you too will feel good! The goal is emotional well-being for you both.

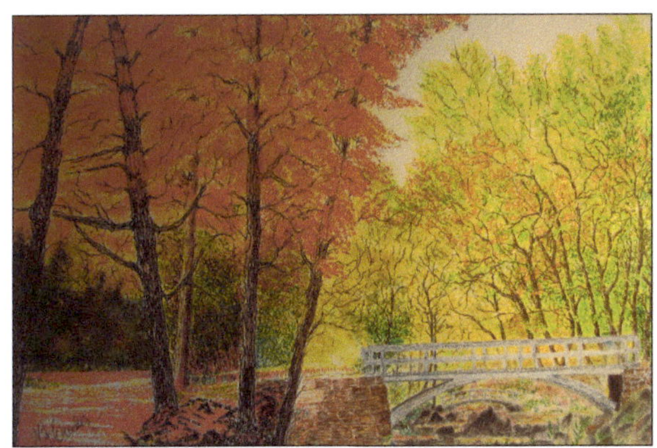

Landscape
Ink Drawing, 2015 • Michael Crookes

Care Partner Distress

Caring about someone living with dementia can play havoc on your emotions. You can't visually see the brain changes to have a sense of what is happening or when there is a change. Most forms of dementia are degenerative, meaning that brain changes and impairments are not singular events but rather ongoing events that occur without warning. These unknowns can cause you (and them) to feel frustrated, angry, upset, fearful, and fatigued among other emotions. Sometimes emotions spill over. One care partner described throwing balled socks when she got upset and frustrated. Another yelled. Another crawled into bed. Dementia causes frustrations and challenges, so it's important to be candid and realistic that there will be times you will need to vent. In fact, safe venting can be a helpful way to release emotions.

The operative word is safe venting. Throwing balled socks is fine, but throwing heavy or breakable objects is not. Mrs. T, a spouse care partner, would use a swear word when really upset. She ordinarily didn't swear, so it not only was a release for her but a signal to her husband. He understood a swear word meant he needed to give her space and time.

Find useful and safe ways to vent while the person experiences mild to moderate symptoms of dementia. It will be a valuable tool for you to use should the dementia symptoms become more advanced and challenging. Mrs. T recounts that during the later stages of her husband's dementia, if she swore he would look so startled that it made her laugh which, in turn, made him laugh.

Behavioral Expressions: Signals of Distress

As noted earlier, distressed behaviors such as frustration, fear, sadness, anger, and denial among others are a normal and natural response to life altering changes experienced by individuals living with dementia. As a care partner it is important to understand what the distressed behaviors signal. If you focus your observational skills, you'll start to understand what triggers what type of distress response. All distressed behaviors have meaning.

The distress with early to moderate symptoms of dementia is often the result of them feeling frustrated and upset when experiencing difficulty doing things that used to come naturally such as concentrating, word-finding, or problem-solving. The distress experienced with advanced symptoms of dementia can be more complex. Since this handbook focuses on early to moderate symptoms of dementia, information about distress experienced in advanced stages are not included here.

Suggestions

- ◆ Depending on the form of dementia, individuals can lose the cognitive ability to self-initiate activities and tasks. While it may appear that they are not interested in doing an activity or task, it is highly possible they don't know how to initiate it. Gently asking whether they need a little help getting started with something can be a caring way to support them without diminishing their self-worth.

◆ Neural damage to the brain that impairs the ability to self-initiate activities can result in the individual becoming inactive and bored. Distressed behaviors can signal the need for support getting them involved in an interesting activity or to go out. A physiological response triggers in the brain when a person is meaningfully engaged and emotionally connected. Naturally produced brain chemicals known as neurotransmitters, such as endorphins, oxytocin, and serotonin, are released into the body. These neurotransmitters produce good feelings and a sense of well-being. The opposite outcome can occur when people are not well supported emotionally. When an individual is bored, fearful, lonely, and inactive the body produces different neurotransmitters, such as cortisol, adrenaline, and norepinephrine. These neurotransmitters serve as important protective measures when, for instance, a hand touches something hot, but they are not beneficial for everyday life. Anyone can successfully support meaningful engagement with a little effort. The more you do it, the better you will get. Staying meaningfully engaged and emotionally connected are essential for well-being.

◆ Depending on the person and form of dementia, some individuals may become hypersensitive to sounds and loud noises. Crowds and people talking while music is playing or a TV is on can sound jarring to them. Be mindful of this dynamic and if a place becomes too noisy, adjust the noise if possible. If adjusting the noise isn't possible, leave or find another place to go. One couple only goes to the shopping center early in the morning because that's when there are the least amount of customers and commotion.

♦ If leaving a noisy place, such as a doctor's office, isn't an option, bring noise cancelling headphones for them. They can listen to some favorite music or just enjoy the quiet.

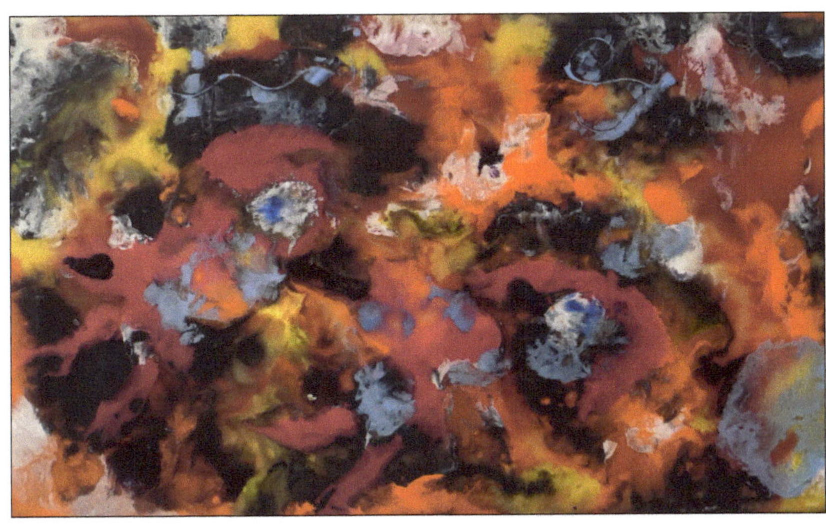

Clash Bang
Encaustic, 2016 • Mandy Looney

Communication Supports

Since individuals with dementia experience difficulty finding words and communicating verbally, it's important to know how to best support the individual's communication abilities. There is a difference between expressive speech (expressing oneself) and receptive speech (understanding what others are saying). Expressive speech abilities can become incrementally impaired with dementia. For most individuals, receptive speech abilities remain functional after expressive speech becomes impaired.

Care partners often mistakenly think that if the individual has difficultly expressing him or herself, they also don't understand what is said. They generally are still able to understand what is being said, but need you to slow down the rate of your speech so their brain can have the extra time to process what is being said.

Stand in front of the individual at their eye level so they can see you while you speak. Seeing your facial expression and lip movements are helpful visual cues.

Suggestions

♦ When word-finding and verbal communication abilities are impaired, it can be challenging to communicate what they want to express. Ask them how you can best support them when this happens. Some individuals want additional time to come up with the words, while others prefer you to offer some word suggestions. Asking how they want to handle this supports their decision-making control which is important for preserving dignity and personhood.

◆ Use short, simple sentences. They are easier to process.

◆ Be pleasant and relaxed when you speak. Your mood and attitude are contagious.

◆ Framing single questions is helpful rather than a statement containing several questions.

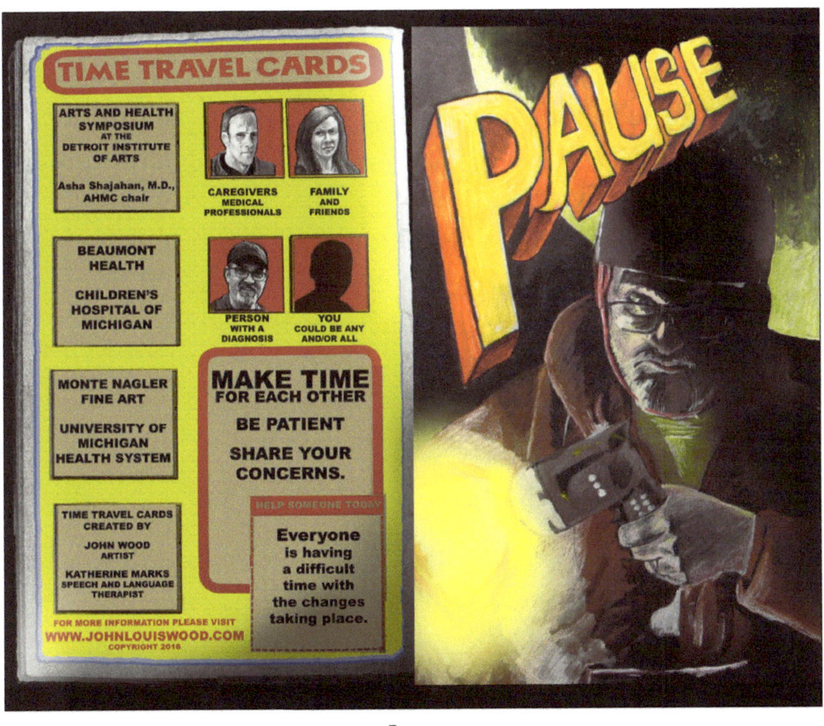

Pause
Illustration, 2016 • John Wood

Holidays and Special Occasions Together

Time with extended family and friends offers precious opportunities to connect and make new memories together. However, these events may be overwhelming for a person living with dementia and stressful for you as well. Holidays and special occasions such as birthdays and anniversaries typically involve more people, lots of activities, and higher noise levels; all of which may be overwhelming to the person living with dementia.

> *"It is easy to feel lonely and isolated in a group of people."*
>
> — Kate Swaffer, with permission

Kate movingly describes what a holiday can feel like to her; the difficulty following conversations and not being able to remember all the things that are being reminisced about. For Kate and others living with dementia, managing a special occasion can be overwhelming. All the sights, sounds, and activities can make a person feel lonely, even though they are surrounded by family and friends who love and care about them. For family and friends, these gatherings can also be stressful. By realizing that some adjustments need to be made, special events can be enjoyable and memorable for everyone.

Sometimes an out-of-town family member or friend who does not often see the individual with dementia may make a comment that, "She or He is doing much better than I expected." While that may feel upsetting to you who has been providing the lion's share of support, realize that sometimes the person living with dementia can function slightly better than usual. The extra love and attention during special occasions can trigger the release of the "feel good" neurotransmitters which can temporarily enhance neural brain connections. With some thoughtful planning and sensitivity to these dynamics, special occasions can be enjoyable for everyone.

> *"This has been our most delightful visit with (my mother) in years, not because she changed, but because we did."*
>
> — Family member working with Dr. Sabat[6]

Suggestions

♦ All the noise and activity can easily become overwhelming for the individual with dementia. Observe the individual during the get-together for signs they are becoming overstimulated or having difficulty managing all the people, noise and activity. If he or she is having difficulty, find a quiet space they can sit. Family and friends can visit one-on-one or with a few others there.

♦ Share the **Communication Supports** information (page 30) with family members and friends in advance so they can be prepared and supportive for communication.

[6] Sabat, S.R. (2012). *A bio-psycho-social model enhances young adults' understanding of and beliefs about people with Alzheimer's disease: A case study.* Dementia: The International Journal of Social Research and Practice, 11:95-112.

♦ Think of a few things you can talk about or do ahead of
time that are special and meaningful to the individual with
dementia. A former gardener, for example, loved it when
her daughter showed photos of her gardens and roses.
Her daughter always mentioned the gift her mother had
for growing beautiful flowers. This never failed to bring
a smile and sense of self-worth to her mother.

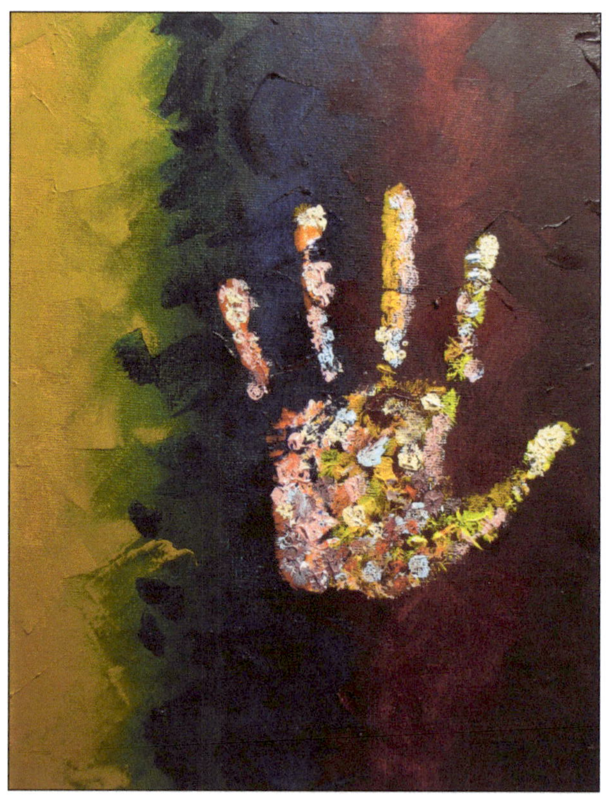

Hand
Acrylic on canvas, 2016 • Maria Nightingale

Final Note

Hopefully this handbook has enhanced your understanding and perspective about someone you care about who is living with dementia. Please visit the Dementia Action Alliance's Resources Center to find other helpful resources including short videos — http://daanow.org/resource-center/.

> *"Try to be a rainbow in someone's cloud."*
>
> — Maya Angelou

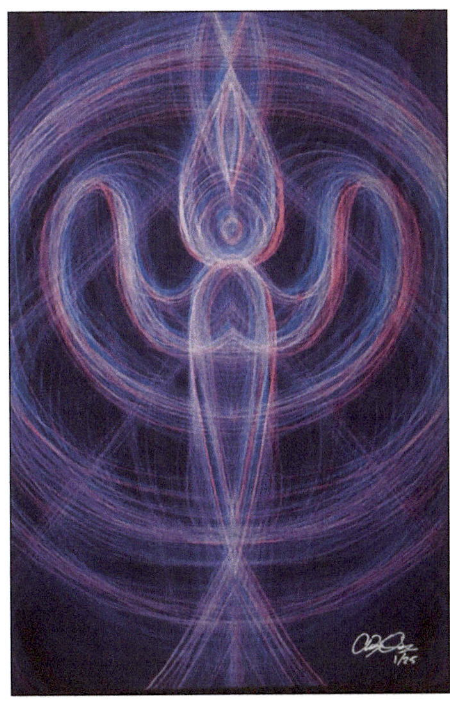

Soul
Digital painting • Chris Deshaine

Resources

The Dementia Action Alliance's website maintains an extensive list of helpful resources including blogs, books, Facebook pages, publications, research centers, video clips and websites from around the world. Please visit http://danow.org/resource-center/.

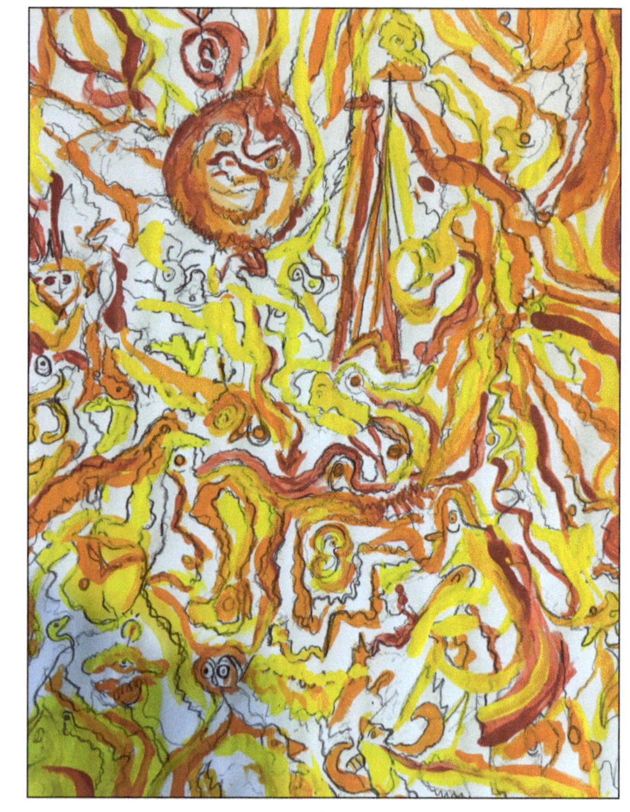

Red Hot
Mixed media • Chris Deshaine

About the Dementia Action Alliance

DAA's Vision

The Dementia Action Alliance (DAA) envisions a society where dementia symptoms are better understood and accommodated as a disability, and individuals and families living with dementia are fully included and supported.

DAA's Mission

The Dementia Action Alliance is a diverse coalition of passionate people creating a better society now for individuals to LIVE with dementia.

DAA's Goals

- WORK directly with individuals who have dementia to learn from and amplify their first person perspectives about dementia.

- EDUCATE the public about living with dementia to raise awareness and increase understanding. Lack of information fosters misperceptions and stigmatizing behaviors toward individuals with dementia.

- COLLABORATE with the diverse dementia community for collective impact to advocate for public policies, practices, and research that optimizes the well-being of people living with dementia.

- CREATE, curate and post free person-centered dementia support resource materials online.

- SUSTAIN the operation of the Dementia Action Alliance.

The Artwork

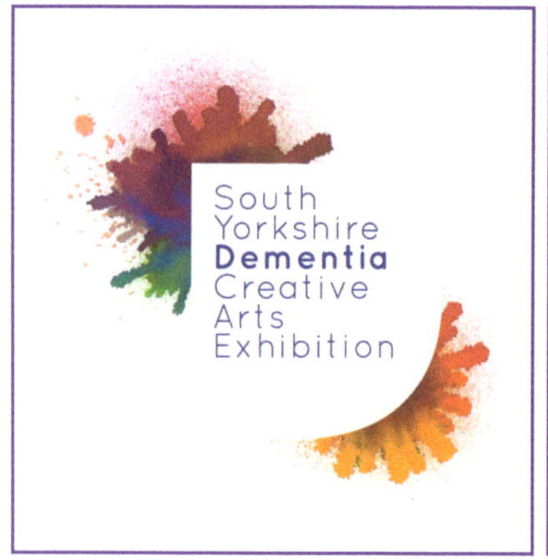
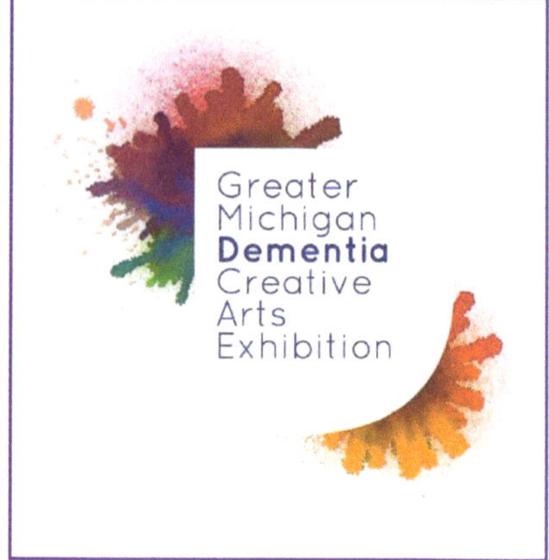

The inspirational artwork throughout the handbook are part of a unique collaborative effort of **David Reid**, Senior University Teacher at the University of Sheffield, England and **John Wood**, a visual artist living with dementia in Detroit, Michigan. David, as part of The University of Sheffield's 'Engaged Learning,' strand of community partnership work, established the South Yorkshire Dementia Creative Arts Exhibition eight years ago. The exhibition features works by individuals who are living with dementia and their care partners to enhance public understanding about life lived with dementia. The exhibition has inspired others and now travels internationally.

John was one of the people inspired by the South Yorkshire Exhibition. Working with others, John created the Greater Michigan Dementia Creative Arts Exhibition in 2015. "Our goal for the exhibition is to be inclusive to all persons involved in a dementia diagnosis. Hopefully the artworks can remove the stigma related to lives affected by dementia.

Meet the Artists

Collaborative – UK **"Blossom Tree"** [care partner]

"This artwork was created by the residents of SheffCare's Springwood Residential Home in Sheffield during our weekly craft sessions. The residents used their hand prints to create branches of our Blossom Tree giving this piece a sense of identity." ~ Sarah Simmonite, Arts Coordinator

Michael Crookes – UK **"Landscape"** [person with dementia]

"Michael uses all types of materials in his artwork, except oils. He currently runs art classes in his local area of Crookes. Michael is inspired by things he sees around him and always carries a pencil and paper with him — ready to sketch."

Chris Deshaine – USA **"Red Hot"** [person with dementia]

I was diagnosed with Alzheimer's disease in my 40's. My artwork helps me focus. I paint every day. I try to work in response to music and let the art flow.

Chris Deshaine – USA **"Soul"** [person with dementia]

See above.

Mandy Looney – USA **"Clash Bang"** [care partner]

My Dad has good days and bad. On the good days I try to find ways to keep his mind active and learn new things.

Maria Nightingale – UK **"Hand"** [care partner/nurse]

The blend of colours is supposed to represent feelings from first diagnosis to the end. When I was painting it, I was thinking of everybody, the person with dementia, their carer and their loved ones. The hand signifies that the simple act of touch is powerful and can bring out happiness in darkness.

Carol Ambrogio Wood – USA **"Garden Tree"** [care partner]

Making art was a break from our daily routine, especially from the stress of dealing with my husband's dementia. It's important to experience new things together, creating new, positive memories.

John Wood – USA **"Pause"** [person with dementia]

I have problems with my memory and communicating. I created with my speech therapist, Katherine Marks, the 'Time Traveller' series of cards to identify specific issues I face when trying to communicate. I share the cards with friends and family when I am struggling. Website — www.johnlouiswood.com .

www.ingramcontent.com/pod-product-compliance
Lightning Source LLC
Chambersburg PA
CBHW040242240726
48664CB00001B/237